Collaborative framework for care and control of tuberculosis and diabetes

Stop TB Department and
Department of Chronic Diseases and Health Promotion
World Health Organization, Geneva, Switzerland

and

The International Union Against Tuberculosis and Lung Disease, Paris, France

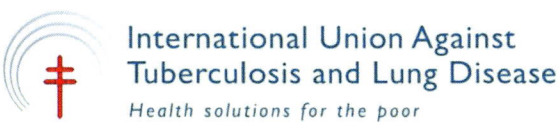

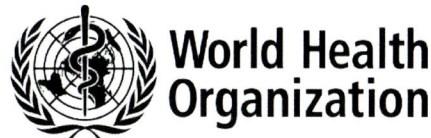

Collaborative framework for care and control of tuberculosis and diabetes.

WHO/HTM/TB/2011.15

1.Tuberculosis - prevention and control. 2.Tuberculosis - etiology. 3.Tuberculosis - complications. 4.Diabetes complications. 4.Diabetes mellitus - prevention and control. 5.Health programs and plans. 6.Guidelines. I.World Health Organization. II.International Union against Tuberculosis and Lung Disease

ISBN 978 92 4 150225 2   (NLM classification: WF 200)

Provisional collaborative framework, 2011

Expiry date, 2015

© World Health Organization 2011

All rights reserved. Publications of the World Health Organization are available on the WHO web site (www.who.int) or can be purchased from WHO Press, World Health Organization, 20 Avenue Appia, 1211 Geneva 27, Switzerland (tel.: +41 22 791 3264; fax: +41 22 791 4857; e-mail: bookorders@who.int).
Requests for permission to reproduce or translate WHO publications – whether for sale or for noncommercial distribution – should be addressed to WHO Press through the WHO web site (http://www.who.int/about/licensing/copyright_form/en/index.html).

The designations employed and the presentation of the material in this publication do not imply the expression of any opinion whatsoever on the part of the World Health Organization concerning the legal status of any country, territory, city or area or of its authorities, or concerning the delimitation of its frontiers or boundaries. Dotted lines on maps represent approximate border lines for which there may not yet be full agreement.

The mention of specific companies or of certain manufacturers' products does not imply that they are endorsed or recommended by the World Health Organization in preference to others of a similar nature that are not mentioned. Errors and omissions excepted, the names of proprietary products are distinguished by initial capital letters.

All reasonable precautions have been taken by the World Health Organization to verify the information contained in this publication. However, the published material is being distributed without warranty of any kind, either expressed or implied. The responsibility for the interpretation and use of the material lies with the reader. In no event shall the World Health Organization be liable for damages arising from its use.

Printed by the WHO Document Production Services, Geneva, Switzerland

Contents

Acknowledgements	iv
Abbreviations	v
Executive summary	vii
1. Introduction	1
1.1 Rationale	1
1.2 Purpose	3
1.3 Target audience	5
2. Framework development process	7
3. Recommended collaborative activities for prevention and care of diabetes and tuberculosis	13
A. Establish mechanisms for collaboration	14
B. Detect and manage tuberculosis in patients with diabetes	19
C. Detect and manage diabetes in patients with tuberculosis	23
4. Indicators for evaluating collaborative activities	26
5. Implementing collaborative activities and evaluating their impact	27
Annexes	28
Annex I. Members of the Guideline Group	28
Annex II. Summary grading of the evidence	30
Annex III. Key research questions for improving prevention, management and care of diabetes and tuberculosis	34
References	35

Support material on the web: Detailed summary of studies included in the systematic reviews (http://www.who.int/tb/publications/2011/en/index.html)
1. Associations between diabetes and tuberculosis infection, tuberculosis disease and drug-resistant tuberculosis
2. Associations between diabetes and tuberculosis treatment outcomes
3. Summary of studies on screening for tuberculosis in diabetes patients and screening for diabetes in tuberculosis patients, and studies on tuberculosis preventive therapy in patients with diabetes

Acknowledgements

The development of this framework was coordinated by Anthony D. Harries and Knut Lönnroth, who also wrote the first draft. The Guideline Group also consisted of (in alphabetical order): Meghan A Baker, Mauricio Barreto, Nils Billo, Richard Brostrom, Ib Christian Bygbjerg, Martin Castellanos, Saidi Egwaga, Susan Fisher-Hoch, Christie Y. Jeon, Megan B. Murray, Toru Mori, Salah-Eddine Ottmani, Kaushik Ramaiya, Gojka Roglic, Nigel Unwin, Vijay Viswanathan, David Whiting, Lixia Wang and Wenhua Zhao. Annex I lists the professional affiliation and area of technical expertise for each group member.

Declaration of conflict of interests

Dr Vijay Viswanathan declared that he had received financial support for consulting and research within the past three years from the World Diabetes Foundation for a project on preventing diabetes among TB patients. No other member of the group reported any conflicts of interest. Individuals affiliated with the World Diabetes Foundation who attended the expert meeting were not engaged in developing this provisional framework.

Review by date

This provisional collaborative framework is due for revision by 2015.

Abbreviations

DOTS	the basic package that underpins the Stop TB Strategy
HbA1c	glycated haemoglobin
HIV	human immunodeficiency virus
NTP	national tuberculosis control programme
OGTT	oral glucose tolerance test
OR	odds ratio
PHC	primary health care
R	rifampicin
RR	relative risk
TB	tuberculosis
The Union	International Union Against Tuberculosis and Lung Disease
WDF	World Diabetes Foundation
WHO	World Health Organization

Executive summary

Diabetes triples the risk of developing tuberculosis (TB). Consequently, rates of TB are higher in people with diabetes than in the general population, and diabetes is a common comorbidity in people with TB. Diabetes can worsen the clinical course of TB, and TB can worsen glycaemic control in people with diabetes. Individuals with both conditions thus require careful clinical management. Strategies are needed to ensure that optimal care is provided to patients with both diseases: TB must be diagnosed early in people with diabetes, and diabetes must be diagnosed early in people with TB.

Changes in lifestyle and diet have contributed to an increased prevalence of diabetes in many low-income and middle-income countries where the burden of TB is high. The growing burden of diabetes is contributing to sustained high levels of TB in the community, and the proportion of TB cases attributable to diabetes globally is likely to increase over time. This double burden of disease is a serious and growing challenge for health systems.

Given the absence of international guidelines on the joint management and control of TB and diabetes, the World Health Organization (WHO) and the International Union Against Tuberculosis and Lung Disease (the Union) identified key questions to be answered and commissioned systematic reviews of studies addressing those questions. A series of expert consultations were organized to assess the findings of the systematic reviews and a guideline group was established to develop this provisional collaborative framework.

The framework aims to guide national programmes, clinicians and others engaged in care of patients and prevention and control of diabetes and TB on how to establish a coordinated response to both diseases, at organizational and clinical levels. The framework is based on evidence collated from systematic reviews and existing guidelines on the diagnosis and management of TB and diabetes. The systematic reviews confirmed the weak evidence base for the effectiveness and cost-effectiveness of collaborative interventions. The framework is therefore provisional; several of its recommendations are provisional pending better evidence. In order to provide advice on how to fill the knowledge gaps, the framework includes a list of priority research areas.

The framework includes the following provisional recommendations:

Establish mechanisms for collaboration
1. Joint coordination should be established at regional, district and/or local levels (sensitive to country-specific factors), with representation from all relevant stakeholders. A joint plan for activities should be drawn up and reflected in national plans for noncommunicable diseases and TB.

2. Surveillance of TB should be initiated among diabetes patients in settings with medium to high burdens of TB.

3. Surveillance of diabetes should be initiated among TB patients in all countries.

4. Where collaborative activities are being established, national programmes should agree a core set of indicators and tools to collect data for monitoring and evaluating activities to improve care and prevention of both diseases. Diabetes programmes should explore the possibility of adapting the DOTS system to monitor and report diabetes cases and treatment outcomes.

Detect and manage TB in patients with diabetes
5. At a minimum, people with diabetes should be screened for chronic cough (that is, cough lasting more than 2 weeks) at the time of their diagnosis with diabetes and, if possible, during regular check-ups. Those with positive TB symptoms should be examined as per national guidelines. Other diagnostic procedures (for example, for extrapulmonary TB) should also be pursued rigorously as per national guidelines.

6. Screening for TB diseases on broader indications (for example, for all people in whom diabetes is diagnosed, regardless of symptoms) should be explored as part of the research agenda to improve the diagnosis of TB among people with diabetes.

7. A referral system should be established so that patients suspected of having TB are promptly referred to TB diagnostic and treatment centres, and evaluated in accordance with guidelines of the national TB control programme.

8. Case-finding for TB should be intensified by increasing awareness of and knowledge about the interactions between diabetes and TB, including joint risk factors, among health-care workers and the populations they serve.

9. Health-care facilities, including diabetes clinics, should have in place an infection control plan that includes administrative and environmental control measures to reduce transmission of TB within health-care settings. These measures should adhere to WHO's international guidelines for TB infection control.

10. Treatment and case management of TB in people with diabetes should be provided in accordance with existing TB treatment guidelines and international standards. The same TB treatment regimen should be prescribed for people with diabetes as for people without diabetes.

Detect and manage diabetes in patients with TB

11. Patients with TB should be screened for diabetes at the start of their treatment, where resources for diagnosis are available. The type of screening and diagnostic tests should be adapted to the context of local health systems and the availability of resources, while awaiting additional evidence on the best screening and diagnostic approach or approaches.

12. Management of diabetes in TB patients should be provided in line with existing management guidelines.

1. Introduction

1.1 Rationale

Intersecting epidemics

Tuberculosis (TB) remains a considerable global public health concern, mainly affecting poor and vulnerable populations (*1*). Every year, more than 9 million people fall ill with this infectious disease, and close to 2 million die from it (*1*). Diabetes, a chronic metabolic disease that is increasing globally, including in many settings with a high burden of TB, is associated with higher risks of TB (*2*) and adverse TB treatment outcomes (*3*). The increase in the number of people with diabetes may further complicate care and control of TB, especially in the many areas with high burden of both diseases (*4, 5*).

In 2010, WHO estimated that 285 million people were living with diabetes, of whom 7 million people developed the disease during that year and 3.9 million deaths were attributed to diabetes (*6, 7*). Current predictions estimate that the prevalence of diabetes will reach 438 million by 2030 and that 80% of prevalent cases will occur in the developing world (*7*). The increase is mainly driven by changes in diet and levels of physical activity (*8*). In the poorest countries, diabetes is more common among the better-off, but economic development quickly reverses this trend so that people from lower socioeconomic groups are more affected by diabetes; sequelae are worse among the poor in all countries (*9*). People from lower socioeconomic groups are therefore more vulnerable to both diseases (*10*).

Mutual risk factors

Intensified discussions and research over the past decade have focused on the links between TB and diabetes (*11, 12*). Many hypotheses have been postulated; the evidence base has grown for some but remains incomplete. Theoretically, diabetes and TB may complicate each other at many levels. Conceivably, people with diabetes may be more easily infected than non-diabetic people leading to a higher risk of latent TB infection, but the evidence remains weak (*13, 14*). TB infection may progress at a faster rate in people with diabetes than in those without diabetes (*2, 15, 16*). The clinical presentation of TB in people with diabetes may be altered and change the sensitivity and specificity of conventional diagnostic algorithms. Among those with active TB, diabetes may adversely affect TB treatment outcomes by delaying the time to microbiological response, reducing the likelihood of a favourable outcome, and increasing the risk of relapse or death (*3*). Diabetes may also accelerate the emergence of drug-resistant TB, especially multidrug-resistant TB (defined as strains of TB resistant to both rifampicin and isoniazid) among those receiving TB treatment, although the evidence is limited (*17*). Conversely, TB may trigger the onset of diabetes, and worsen glycaemic control in existing diabetes. Finally, TB medications may interfere with the treatment of diabetes through drug interactions, and diabetes may interfere with the activity of certain anti-TB medicines (*18*).

Gaps in care and control of TB

Over the past two decades, national TB control programmes worldwide have implemented TB control through DOTS and the Stop TB Strategy with evident success, including substantial increases in rates of case detection and improved treatment outcomes (*1*). However, improvements are still needed to tackle the following challenges:

First, countries must ensure complete and early case detection of all types of TB. During 2005–2009, the global TB case detection rate stagnated at around 60% (*19*). In many countries these rates are even lower, and long delays for diagnosis and treatment still occur in most countries (*20*), further aggravating transmission. Case detection of smear-negative TB and for multidrug resistant-TB also must be substantially improved (*1*).

Second, while the rate of treatment success globally has surpassed the target of 85%, treatment outcomes are suboptimal in many settings and for some subpopulations (*1*). Where adverse treatment outcomes are frequent, reasons may include poor adherence to treatment, high prevalence of drug-resistance and/or vulnerability related to co-morbidities such as HIV, under-nutrition, substance dependency, tobacco smoking-related conditions and diabetes.

Third, although rates of incidence, prevalence and death from TB are decreasing globally, the rate of decline is much slower than forecast (*1*). Given this slow rate of decline, the Millennium Development Goal target of halving TB prevalence and TB death rates by 2015, compared with their levels in 1990, may not be met in all WHO regions. Furthermore, the world as a whole, as well as in most regions, are far from the trend required to reach the long-term rates of eliminating TB (defined as less than 1 incident case of TB per one million population by 2050) (*1*). Additional interventions are therefore required to meet the goals for TB control and elimination. Most urgently, this should involve further efforts to improve TB case detection and treatment outcomes, with the ultimate aim to get as close as possible to 100%

case detection rate and treatment success rate. Moreover, new tools for TB diagnosis, prevention and treatment are needed. Additional efforts should also include prevention by intervening on known social determinants and risk factors of TB, such as HIV/AIDS, smoking, malnutrition, alcohol dependency, diabetes, crowded living conditions, and indoor air pollution to reduce people's vulnerability to TB disease (*1, 21*).

Synergies of collaborative activities
The link between diabetes and TB has potential additional implications for all the above-mentioned challenges to TB control. First, given that people with diabetes are at higher risk of TB, screening for TB in people with diabetes may be warranted in populations with high TB prevalence to help improve early case detection. Second, because diabetes may increase the risk of adverse treatment outcomes in TB patients, special attention may be needed to ensure high-quality TB treatment in people with diabetes. This requires screening for diabetes among people with TB in settings where under-diagnosis of diabetes is common. Third, broad primary and secondary prevention of diabetes will help prevent TB at the population level. Finally, TB preventive therapy could potentially be indicated in people with diabetes who have had recent exposure to TB.

Improved collaborative activities would also potentially improve care and prevention of diabetes. Under-diagnosis of the disease is common in low-income and middle income countries, and could be improved by screening people with TB for diabetes. Management of diabetes must be optimized in general, and in particular during TB disease, as during all types of infections. Improved management of diabetes could build on the successes of the DOTS strategy, emphasizing support to patients and supervision of their treatment; standardized protocols, a reliable supply of quality-assured medicines, regular monitoring and evaluation, and management and administrative procedures; as well as political commitment.

1.2 Purpose of the collaborative framework

The purpose of the collaborative framework is to assist policy-makers, public health practitioners and clinicians in understanding how to decrease the joint burden of diabetes and TB. It responds to a growing concern about what collaborative activities should be implemented and under what circumstances. The framework is complementary to and in synergy with the established core activities of prevention and care programmes for both diseases. The *Stop TB Strategy* (*22*) and the *International Standards for Tuberculosis Care* (*23*) set out the key elements of TB care and control. Similarly, a set of activities to prevent, diagnose and treat diabetes form the basis of strategies to control diabetes (24).

The framework does not call for the institution of a new specialist or independent control programme. Rather, it promotes enhanced collaboration between diabetes and TB prevention and care programmes with the overall aim of improving collaboration between disease control programmes, as a part of the broader agenda for strengthening health systems. Effective collaboration between TB and HIV/AIDS programmes during the past decades has helped avoid unnecessary duplication of service delivery structures, and has promoted optimal and well-coordinated use of scarce health-care resources. The proposed framework builds on the experience of TB/HIV collaboration, and applies its key elements to TB and diabetes. The elements could also be further applied to other risk factors for TB and associated co-morbidities. WHO and its partners are reviewing the impact of other TB risk factors and co-morbidities, such as tobacco smoking-related conditions (25), under-nutrition (26), alcohol dependency (27) and substance abuse (28).

Ideally, a future collaborative framework should encompass coordination across all relevant programmes for infectious and noncommunicable diseases. However, the evidence base is still not strong enough for such a comprehensive framework.

Scientific evidence of the links between TB and diabetes is also incomplete for certain aspects of the interaction, and there are insufficient data to support specific guidance on several key elements of collaborative activities. Given the lack of high-quality evidence, the framework does not include any recommendations on diagnosis of latent TB infection and preventive treatment of latent TB infection in people with diabetes. Nevertheless, sufficient evidence exists to formulate a set of broad recommendations, which would have to be fine-tuned as more evidence becomes available.

For these reasons, the framework is provisional in nature, with existing evidence from observational studies being used to support policy recommendations. It is a rolling framework, which will be updated to reflect new evidence and best practices. It should be reviewed and revised by 2015. The framework is intended to help stimulate operational research. As better scientific evidence and documented country experiences become available, this framework should be further developed into global policy and guidelines for collaborative activities.

1.3 Target audience

This document is intended for decision-makers and public health practitioners (including managers of national TB control programmes, and initiatives for care and prevention of diabetes), as well as development agencies, nongovernmental organizations, researchers and funding agencies in the field of public health and disease control. The recommendations made in this document may have important implications for the strategic directions and activities of other ministries. The document also targets, indirectly, clinicians working at all levels of the health sector. However, the framework will need national and local adaptation, including development of national clinical guidance, as part of guidelines on TB and diabetes respectively.

The recommendations may not be equally relevant in all countries. The relative importance of pursuing collaborative activities depends on the national or local context, including the prevalence of both diseases, the availability of diagnostic and treatment services for diabetes, the strength of national TB control programmes, competing priority areas and availability of resources. The document may therefore be most relevant in countries with high TB burdens and high or rapidly increasing prevalence of diabetes.

Strong national TB control programmes and programmes for the prevention and care of diabetes are ideal starting points to implement this framework. Where such programmes already exist, the key actions are ensuring coordination between programmes, introducing basic screening approaches across both programmes, and initiating effective cross-referral between services. Where both services are available within the same primary health-care structure, such coordination should be relatively straightforward. The exact division of roles between services will depend on the country context. In principle, however, it should be possible to do basic screening for diabetes among people with TB (for example, with random blood glucose) in a TB facility, and to do simple symptom screening for TB in diabetes clinics, and refer for TB diagnostic tests as required. TB treatment should in most situations be initiated in a TB facility, although the continuous treatment support and supervision can be done in any facility. All parts of diabetes management may not necessarily be done in a diabetes facility. For example, health education and advice on self-management of treatment may be partly incorporated into the service package that is delivered during the regular health-care contacts that are a part of TB treatment, especially during the directly-observed treatment applied during the intensive phase (first two months), and sometimes beyond.

If services for diabetes are not well developed, as is the case in several high TB burden countries, some of the recommendations in this framework may not be appropriate. Nevertheless, the framework can be used to stimulate collaborative efforts to strengthen diabetes services (as well as services for noncommunicable diseases in general) with a view to creating the necessary conditions for good, comprehensive, patient-centred care, that will benefit both TB care and control, as well as care and prevention for diabetes and other noncommunicable diseases.

2. Framework development process

In January 2009, WHO and the Union organized a meeting at WHO headquarters in Geneva, Switzerland, to review existing evidence and identify priority questions for systematic reviews of the links between diabetes and TB. The meeting prioritized questions to be addressed based on (i) identified gaps in evidence; (ii) relevance of the questions for policy and practice primarily in low-income and middle-income countries with high burdens of TB and high or growing burdens of diabetes; (iii) potential for immediate development of programmatic policy; and (iv) the likelihood that available evidence could be obtained through systematic reviews. The prioritized questions are listed in box 1.

Box 1: Questions addressed through systematic reviews

1. Is diabetes associated with TB infection?
2. Is diabetes associated with active TB disease?
3. Is diabetes associated with positive sputum culture at 2–3 months?
4. Is diabetes associated with favourable TB treatment outcome?
5. Is diabetes associated with death during treatment period?
6. Is diabetes associated with recurrent TB disease?
7. Is diabetes associated with TB drug-resistance?
8. Does screening for TB among people with diabetes lead to more TB case detection?
9. Does screening for diabetes among TB patients lead to more diabetes detection?
10. Does hyperglycaemia initially found in TB patients resolve with TB treatment?
11. Is chemoprophylaxis in diabetes effective in preventing TB?
12. Does screening for TB among people with diabetes lead to better prevention of TB morbidity and mortality compared with no screening?
13. Does screening for diabetes among TB patients lead to better prevention of diabetes morbidity and mortality compared with no screening?

The systematic reviews of the literature were commissioned from the Harvard School of Public Health, USA, which had previously published a systematic review addressing question 2: is diabetes associated with active TB disease? (2). An updated review was conducted on the association of diabetes and TB disease; new reviews were conducted to address the other questions. Studies were searched for in (i) PubMed (from 1965 to June 2009); (ii) in EMBASE (from 1974 to June 2009); and (iii) conference proceedings of the Union (for 2007 and 2008).

For the aims of identifying studies on the association between diabetes and TB infection, the full text of studies including any of the following terms related to TB infection in the abstract were examined: "latent", OR "tuberculin skin", OR "PPD", OR "interferon" OR "Mantoux" OR "Heaf" OR "Tine". Any study quantifying the association between diabetes and TB infection, or allowing the computation of a relative risk, were included in the final analysis. To identify studies on the association between diabetes and TB, studies measuring the effect of risk factors for active TB in full text were scanned to determine if diabetes had been included as a risk factor. Studies measuring the association between diabetes and TB after adjusting for age were included in the systematic review, as they had been for the previously published systematic review (2).

In order to identify studies on the association of diabetes and drug-resistant TB, studies including any of the following terms in the abstract were examined: "drug-resistant", "drug-resistance", "multidrug-resistant", "drug resistant" or "drug resistance", "MDR TB" or "MDRTB". The full text of studies examining risk factors for drug-resistant TB was scanned to determine whether diabetes had been assessed as a risk factor for TB. Studies that quantified the association between diabetes and drug-resistant TB, or that allowed the computation of a relative risk, were included.

To identify studies on the association between diabetes and TB treatment outcomes, studies on diabetes and TB were searched for, as well as studies on TB outcomes not necessarily mentioning diabetes in the abstract. Studies providing or permitting the computation of an effect estimate of the relationship between diabetes and at least one of the following five TB treatment outcomes were included: (i) proportion of treated patients with culture conversion at 2–3 months; (ii) the combined outcome of treatment failure and death; (iii) death; (iv) relapse; (v) or recurrent drug-resistant TB. For the aims of summarizing studies on TB outcomes, the literature search was expanded to include the WHO Regional Indexes (AIM (AFRO), LILACS (AMRO/PAHO), IMEMR (EMRO), IMSEAR (SEARO), WPRIM (WPRO)) (http://www.globalhealthlibrary.net/php/index.php) and extended to 31

December 2010 at the request of reviewers considering the systematic review for publication.

To address whether screening for TB in people with diabetes or screening for diabetes in people with TB will lead to detection of new cases, studies that included any of the following root terms in the abstract: "screen*", "detect*", "diagnos*", "chemoproph*", "isoniazid*" and "prevent*" were searched.

    a. To assess the yield of screening for TB disease among diabetics, studies that actively screened a population of previously diagnosed diabetics for active TB using any of the following methods of identification were included: X-ray consistent with TB, positive sputum smear microscopy, positive mycobacterial culture, clinical diagnosis, and response to anti-TB treatment. Studies that did not describe the age distribution of the screened population were excluded.

    b. To assess the yield of screening for diabetes among TB patients, studies were included that screened a population of patients with active TB for diabetes using a blood glucose test, including random blood glucose, fasting blood glucose, oral glucose tolerance test and measurement of haemoglobin A1c. Studies were excluded that did not describe the age distribution of the screened population, and studies that only diagnosed impaired glucose tolerance.

    c. To assess the efficacy of chemoprophylaxis in diabetics, studies that had compared the incidence of TB in a diabetic population receiving TB chemoprophylaxis to a control population also with diabetes were included. The use of any standard anti-TB agent and analogs administered for any duration of time was considered.

For the associations with TB infection and TB disease, the studies were grouped by study design. For the associations with drug-resistant TB, the studies were grouped by type of drug-resistance (any drug-resistance, multidrug-resistance, or extensive drug resistance) and by primary or acquired status. For studies on associations with TB outcomes, separate analyses were performed for each of the outcomes. The heterogeneity of the effect estimates was assessed within these categories by the Cochran Q test and the Higgins I (2) value. For subgroups with no heterogeneity, the findings by fixed effects meta-analysis were summarized. When heterogeneity was present the Dersimonian-Laird random effects meta-analysis was performed. The possibility of publication bias was examined by the Begg and Egger test and by visually inspecting the funnel plot for asymmetry.

Studies on screening for TB among people with diabetes were grouped into those that assessed TB prevalence and those that assessed TB incidence through longitudinal follow-up. The prevalence or the incidence rates of TB found in people with diabetes and controls were calculated where data were available. For follow-up studies, the annual TB incidences were summarized by dividing the cumulative incidence by the number of years of follow-up. For studies that provided the number of TB cases diagnosed by X-ray separately from those diagnosed by bacteriology, the latter definition was used to calculate TB prevalence. Prevalence or incidence ratios and prevalence or incidence differences were computed to assess the relative and absolute contrast in yield of finding TB cases between the screened diabetic populations and the comparison populations where available. Additionally, the number of people needed to screen to detect one additional case of TB in a diabetic population was calculated by taking the inverse of the prevalence or incidence difference for each study.

The systematic reviews were completed by the end of August 2009. The systematic reviews have resulted in peer-reviewed journal papers, which describe the methods and results in detail and provide further information about the reviewed studies (*2, 3, 33*). The main findings from the systematic reviews are summarized in Box 1. Grading of the evidence (*29*) for each respective question is presented in Annex II. Detailed summaries of the studies included in the systematic reviews are provided on the WHO website: http://www.who.int/tb/publications/2011/en/index.html.

Box 2: Summary of findings in the systematic reviews

1. Diabetes is associated with an increased risk of active TB both in case-control studies and in cohort studies. However, there is no evidence to suggest that diabetes increases susceptibility to TB infection. It is not yet fully established that the risk of TB increases with poor glucose control, although this association is plausible, and some indirect evidence supports this hypothesis. Full details are provided in the previously published systematic review (2). The updated review identified three additional studies on the association between diabetes and active TB published between March 2007 and May 2009. In summary, there were four cohort studies where the pooled random effect relative risk of TB in diabetes patients was 2.52 (95% CI 1.53–4.03). There were 10 case-control studies where the odds ratios ranged from 1.16–7.81, with a random effects summary OR of 2.2. There were two studies that stratified diabetes by glycaemic control and showed that higher blood glucose levels were associated with higher risk of TB. Full details of these studies are provided in support material No. 1 at
http://www.who.int/tb/publications/2011/en/index.html

2. Diabetes appears to impact on several key TB treatment outcomes: it may increase the time to sputum culture conversion, and it increases the risk of death and the risk of TB relapse. However, there is no evidence that diabetes increases the risk of recurrence caused by drug-resistant strains. Detailed methodology and summary of reviewed studies are provided in the published systematic review (3). The reasons for these adverse outcomes are not clear. Diabetes may be associated with decreased rifampicin concentrations, which may result from drug–drug interactions between anti-TB drugs and oral hypoglycaemic drugs. DM may also be a risk factor for hepatic toxicity of anti-TB drugs. Thus, lower anti-TB drug concentrations and increased hepatic toxicity may lead to increased recurrent disease and increased death rates respectively. Rifampicin, a known inducer of drug metabolizing enzymes in the liver, consistently decreases pharmacokinetic parameters of multiple oral diabetic agents, and this in turn can impair glucose control. This cumulative evidence suggests that increased attention should be paid to the treatment of TB in people with diabetes, which may include diabetes testing, improved glucose control and increased clinical and therapeutic monitoring. However, there is no evidence from trials assessing the effectiveness and cost-effectiveness of such interventions. Full details of these studies are provided in support material No. 2 at http://www.who.int/tb/publications/2011/en/index.html

3. In screenings studies, TB prevalence and incidence are consistently higher in people with diabetes than in either the general population or in non-diabetic controls. However, the magnitude of this difference varies between countries and there is a very limited evidence base from low-income countries and none at all from sub-Saharan Africa. The burden of TB is higher in people with diabetes who are insulin-dependent compared with those who do not require insulin. The prevalence of diabetes is also higher in TB patients than in healthy controls or the general population, but the data suggest that blood glucose levels fall with TB treatment raising questions about when is the optimal time to screen for diabetes in TB patients on anti-TB treatment. Intensified screening for TB among people with known diabetes would potentially improve early TB case detection, but this approach has rarely been tested under programmatic conditions. The number needed to screen to detect one case of TB varies with underlying TB prevalence. In settings in which TB prevalence is less than 25 per 100 000 persons, at least 1000 people with diabetes would need to be screened, whereas in places with higher TB burden the number needed to screen is considerably lower. For example, in India with an estimated TB prevalence of 283/100 000 people, screening 90 to 350 people with diabetes would yield one or more cases of TB. Detailed methodology and summary of reviewed studies are provided in the published systematic review (33). Full details of the included studies are provided in support material No. 3 at
http://www.who.int/tb/publications/2011/en/index.html

4. There is limited evidence from only two trials done 50 years ago that isoniazid preventive therapy reduces the risk of TB in people with diabetes. However, the trials were poorly conducted and the true benefit and risks of TB preventive therapy in people with diabetes remain unknown. Details are provided in support material No. 3 at http://www.who.int/tb/publications/2011/en/index.html

The findings of the systematic review were presented and assessed at an expert meeting held in November 2009 at The Union in Paris, France. The meeting was attended by experts in the field of diabetes and TB; included were representatives from WHO, The Union, the World Diabetes Foundation, the International Diabetes Federation, academic institutions, and ministries of health in low-income and middle-income countries. The main objectives of the meeting were to assess the results of the systematic reviews and to determine whether there was enough evidence to make policy recommendations about joint diagnosis and management of both diseases, address research gaps and develop a research agenda around these gaps (30). The experts assessed the quality of the systematic reviews, including the search strategy, inclusion/exclusion criteria, and interpretation and presentation of findings. The research agenda is included in Annex III (31). The results of the systematic review as well as the recommendations from the meeting were presented and discussed at the 40th Union World Conference on Lung Health in December 2009.

Following the meeting, it was decided that there was enough evidence from the systematic review and existing guidelines on both diseases to allow a provisional collaborative framework to be developed. The plan to develop a collaborative framework was approved by the WHO Guideline Review Committee, and a guideline group was established (29). The coordinators of the work from WHO and The Union drafted the framework, including specific recommendations. The draft was circulated to all members of the group and discussed in a series of conference calls. Altogether three iterations of the framework and recommendations were circulated to the group members; the final version was approved by all members. There were no major disagreements on the recommendations among the group's members. The recommendations were based in the findings in the systematic reviews, on existing guidelines on TB and DM diagnosis and treatment, and on expert opinions. The recommendations that are based on graded evidence emerging from the systematic reviews have been graded as strong, weak, or conditional. Other recommendations are not graded.

The draft was presented to WHO's Strategic and Technical Advisory Group for TB on 28 September 2010. Several of the group's recommendations were considered in finalizing the provisional framework.

3. Recommended collaborative activities

The goal of the framework is to guide the development and implementation of collaborative activities aimed at decreasing the joint burden of diabetes and TB in populations affected by both diseases. The objectives of those collaborative activities are:

A. To establish mechanisms of collaboration between diabetes and TB programmes;
B. To improve detection and management of TB in patients with diabetes; and
C. To improve detection and management of diabetes in TB patients.

The recommended activities are listed in table 1.

This document focuses on collaborative activities that address the interface of the diabetes and TB epidemics and that should be carried out as part of the health sector's response to this dual disease burden. In all high TB burden countries there is an established national TB control programme, which is the key counterpart for such collaboration, while other local, national and international partners involved in TB care and control should also be involved. National programmes or initiatives for prevention and care of diabetes are generally less developed, at least in low-income and middle income countries with high TB burdens. The counterpart(s) for collaboration may therefore be more difficult to identify, and collaboration may have to start at a local and clinical level while national structures for diabetes prevention and care or for noncommunicable diseases as a group are being developed further.

Table 1: Recommended collaborative activities

A. Establish mechanisms for collaboration

A.1. Set up means of coordinating diabetes and TB activities
A.2. Conduct surveillance of TB disease prevalence among people with diabetes in medium and high-TB burden settings
A.3. Conduct surveillance of diabetes prevalence in TB patients in all countries
A.4. Conduct monitoring and evaluation of collaborative diabetes and TB activities

B. Detect and manage TB in patients with diabetes

B.1. Intensify detection of TB among people with diabetes
B.2. Ensure TB infection control in health-care settings where diabetes is managed
B.3. Ensure high quality TB treatment and management in people with diabetes

C. Detect and manage diabetes in patients with TB

C.1. Screen TB patients for diabetes
C.2. Ensure high-quality diabetes management among TB patients

A. Establish mechanisms for collaboration

A.1. Set up means of coordinating diabetes and TB activities

Few countries have established formal coordination between programmes for prevention and care of diabetes and TB control programmes, although integration of clinical care for both conditions may be in place at the local or clinical level.

A coordinating body should be set up to ensure more effective collaboration between existing programmes. As these cut across the interface between noncommunicable diseases and communicable diseases, such a coordinating body should also consider improved collaboration on other common co-morbidities, such as respiratory illnesses, substance abuse and malnutrition, as well as metabolic problems related to treatment of HIV (32). If such a coordinating body already exists, coordination of activities for both diseases may be incorporated into its terms of reference. The coordinating body should include representatives from relevant Ministry of Health departments, including those responsible for appropriate disease control programmes, hospitals or curative care, national health insurance and private health care regulation, as well as of professional associations, patient groups for both diseases and civil society.

A key area for the joint coordinating bodies is to ensure joint planning between the prevention and care services for diabetes and TB control programmes. The joint plan should be reflected in the plan for noncommunicable diseases including diabetes and the national TB control plan, and encompass:
- development of guidelines and tools for bi-directional screening of TB and diabetes and for treatment and management of the two diseases, including clearly defined roles and responsibilities, and mechanisms for cross-referrals, at national and district levels;
- governance, standards and mechanisms for quality control;
- resource mobilization, including sufficient support for health-care delivery in the field of laboratory, medicines and referral capacity;
- pre-service and in-service training;
- joint advocacy, communication and social mobilization addressing the needs of individual patients and communities for clinical care and prevention of both diseases;
- research, especially operational research, on country-specific issues to develop the evidence base for efficient and effective implementation of collaborative activities.

Mutual advocacy is an essential element of this coordination. National TB control programmes should assist programmes for prevention and care of diabetes to advocate for improved prevention and care, and vice versa, using the existing evidence on the link between the two diseases, and securing translation of new knowledge to best practice.

Recommendation 1
Joint coordination should be established at regional, district and/or local levels (sensitive to country-specific factors), with representation from all relevant stakeholders. A joint plan for diabetes and TB activities should be drawn up and reflected in the national plans on noncommunicable diseases and TB respectively.

Remarks: No published studies on the feasibility and effects of joint coordination of diabetes and TB services have been identified. However the experts in the guideline group judged that this is an essential first step, which would be acceptable and feasible in most settings. Coordination does not necessarily mean additional resources for new infrastructure or manpower. It can be achieved with existing resources, depending on the local situation, and may be a part of coordination mechanisms for TB and other relevant TB co-morbidities, such as HIV, chronic obstructive pulmonary disease and substance dependency.

A.2. Conduct surveillance of prevalence of TB disease in people with diabetes in medium and high-TB burden settings

Data on TB burden among people with diabetes, and vice versa, are available in only a few countries (*33*), from research studies. Surveillance is essential to inform planning and implementation. The two key methods for surveillance of TB in diabetes patients are: (i) periodic (special) cross-sectional surveys among representative groups of diabetes patients within a country; and (ii) data from routine TB screening in diabetes patients. The methods used depend on the prevalence of both diseases in the country and the availability of resources. TB screening should follow the national TB guidelines of the country, although the special surveys may utilize other technologies than the standard screening and diagnostic algorithms specified in such guidelines.

In settings where TB prevalence is low, the number of people with diabetes that needs to be screened to detect one case of TB is very large; therefore, surveillance of TB among people with diabetes may not be relevant and feasible in such settings. The recommendation is therefore to conduct surveillance in settings with an estimated TB prevalence exceeding 100/100 000 population.

Recommendation 2
There should be TB surveillance among diabetes patients in settings with medium to high TB burden.

Remarks: No published studies were identified on the feasibility of TB surveillance among diabetes patients. The experts agreed that such surveillance would be of value in contributing to detection of additional TB cases as well as in providing epidemiological data for decision-making on TB screening among people with diabetes, with no risk of adverse consequences for patients as long as adequate TB treatment resources are available. However, where resources are limited, it may not be feasible to introduce TB surveillance even where prevalence of the disease is high.

A.3. Conduct surveillance of diabetes in TB patients in all countries

Surveillance of diabetes in TB patients may involve (i) periodic (special) cross-sectional surveys among a representative group of TB patients; and/or (ii) data from routine screening for diabetes among TB patients (see section C.1. below). The method depends on the availability of resources and existing structure of the health system and its capacity.

A simple postprandial blood glucose measurement with a glucometer 2 hours after a meal is the preferred method for diagnosing diabetes in primary health-care settings where ease of use, cheapness, speed, reliability and acceptability are paramount. This method will regularly identify more diabetes patients than fasting and/or random blood sugar (FBS/RBS). However, FBS/RBS can also be used, as long as it is understood that sensitivity is lower than for postprandial blood glucose. Measurement of glycated haemoglobin (HbA1c) or the oral glucose tolerance test is effective but expensive and time-consuming. Both assays, particularly the HbA1c, are useful in confirming a glucometer reading (*34*).

In the 22 countries with a high burden of TB, the prevalence of diabetes ranges from 2% to 9% in the general population (*1*). Given the increased risk of TB among people with diabetes, its prevalence among people with TB is generally 2–3 times higher than that of the general population. Therefore, the number of TB patients needed to screen to detect a case of diabetes, as well as sample size required for periodic cross-sectional surveys, is small. Surveillance of diabetes among people with TB should be feasible and affordable in all countries where basic equipment and knowledge of diabetes is available in primary health care.

Recommendation 3
There should be surveillance of diabetes among TB patients in all countries.

Remarks: No published studies were identified on the feasibility of diabetes surveillance among TB patients. However, the guideline group concluded that such surveillance would be beneficial and feasible in most settings. Resource requirements may be modest in most settings since diabetes testing in a relatively small sample of TB patients would likely be sufficient. However, where resources are very limited, it may not be feasible to introduce testing.

A.4. Conduct monitoring and evaluation of collaborative diabetes and TB activities

Monitoring and evaluation provides the means to regularly assess the quality, effectiveness, coverage and delivery of collaborative activities. The DOTS component of the Stop TB Strategy, allows structured, well-monitored services to be delivered to millions of TB patients in some of the poorest countries worldwide. The recommended monitoring strategy for national TB control programmes already includes monitoring and reporting of HIV parameters, and this should similarly include monitoring and reporting of diabetes prevalence among TB patients. Indicators for monitoring collaborative TB and diabetes activities are further discussed in section 4 below.

The concept of using components of the DOTS model to manage diabetes has already been proposed (*35*, *36*), and diabetes clinics in urban areas in high-burden countries may pilot and evaluate this approach through operational research. In particular, diabetes clinics should assess whether quarterly cohort reporting of incident cases, cumulative outcomes, complications and survival analysis can lead to better management and care, and more rational forecasting and uninterrupted supplies of medicines. The monitoring and evaluation of TB cases identified during screening needs to be included into this model.

Recommendation 4
Where diabetes and TB collaboration is being established, programmes for both diseases should agree on a core set of indicators and data collection tools for the monitoring and evaluation of collaborative activities. Diabetes programmes should explore the possibility of adapting the DOTS system to monitor and report cases and treatment outcomes.

Remarks: No published studies on the feasibility and effects of jointly developing indicators for evaluation and monitoring of TB and diabetes were identified. However, many national TB control programmes have used a standard set of key indicators and routine data collection and reporting forms for almost two decades, and their feasibility and utility has been established through regular national, regional and global reporting of TB control activities and results (*19*). Improved management of diabetes could potentially build on the successes of the DOTS strategy, emphasizing regular monitoring and evaluation.

B. Detect and manage TB in patients with diabetes

B.1. Intensify detection of TB among people with diabetes

Early identification of TB symptoms and signs, followed by diagnosis and prompt treatment, increases the chances of survival, improves the quality of life and reduces transmission of TB in the clinic and in the community.

Evidence shows that the prevalence of TB is considerably higher among people with diabetes than in the general population (*18*). Therefore, the current recommendation to screen for TB symptoms and identify people with cough for more than 2–3 weeks should be implemented rigorously in this risk group. In practice, this means that clinicians need to be alert to the presence of cough among people with diabetes, as well as be prepared to ask people with diabetes about cough, at least at the time of their diagnosis, and at regular intervals, for example as a part of routine clinical follow-up. Appropriate referral mechanisms for suspected or confirmed TB need to be put in place, as well as routine systems for recording and reporting, with adequate training of all concerned staff. This should be developed as part of the joint plan for collaborative activities.

There is currently insufficient evidence supporting more active screening approaches, for example, regular screening of all people with diabetes for TB disease using radiography, sputum smear microscopy or other tests, or to conduct these investigations based on the presence of any TB symptom or sign. However, unexplained cough, long-lasting fever and/or other signs or symptoms associated with TB should heighten clinical suspicion of TB in people with diabetes, especially in high TB burden settings. The number needed to screen, and the cost-effectiveness of screening, depends on the prevalence of TB among people with diabetes, the eligibility criteria for screening, and the sensitivity, specificity and cost of the chosen screening and diagnostic approach in the given setting. In settings where it is relevant to pursue more active case detection strategies, and where resources permit, comprehensive screening of people with diabetes should be explored as part of the research agenda for improved TB case detection. Operational research is encouraged to determine (i) the most effective type of screening algorithm; (ii) how often screening should be conducted; and (iii) the most appropriate TB screening tools.

Recommendation 5
At a minimum, people with diabetes should be asked about the presence of cough (lasting more than 2 weeks) at the time of diabetes diagnosis,

and if possible at each regular check-up for diabetes. Those with positive symptoms should be examined as per national guidelines. Other diagnostic procedures, such as those for extrapulmonary TB, should also be pursued rigorously as per national guidelines.

Remark: The evidence for existing guidelines on TB screening and diagnosis was not reviewed as part of the systematic review for this document. However, this recommendation is fully in line with existing guidelines on TB screening and diagnosis (*37*), and should therefore be highly acceptable in most settings. Feasibility and resource implications are the same as for screening of TB symptoms and diagnosis among other groups of patients seeking care with TB symptoms.

Recommendation 6
Screening for active TB on broader indications (for example in all people diagnosed with diabetes, regardless of symptoms) should be explored as part of the research agenda for improved TB diagnosis among people with diabetes.

Summary of assessment of graded evidence from the systematic reviews

Overall quality of evidence	Very low
Balance of potential benefits and harms	Benefit
Disagreement among the panel	None
Acceptability	High
Feasibility	Dependent on setting
Resource implications	High
Strength of recommendation	STRONG

Remark: The direct evidence on screening for active TB among people with diabetes is of very low quality. There are no published studies on the feasibility and additional yield of routinely conducted TB screening among people with diabetes. There are no studies on the impact of increased TB screening among people with diabetes on TB morbidity or mortality. However, there is evidence of moderate quality that diabetes is associated with TB and that its prevalence among people with diabetes is two to three times higher than in the general population. The guideline group agreed to make this a strong recommendation while emphasizing that pursuing such screening is a part of the research agenda.

Recommendation 7
A referral system should be established so that patients with suspected TB are promptly sent to TB diagnostic and treatment centres, and

evaluated in accordance with the Guidelines of the national TB control programme.

Remark: Although no published studies were identified on establishing a referral system between TB and diabetes services, the guideline group's experts agreed that effective referral mechanisms are an essential element of any health-care system.

Recommendation 8
Tuberculosis case-finding should be intensified by increasing the awareness and knowledge of the interactions between diabetes and TB, including joint risk factors, among health-care workers and the populations they serve.

Remark: No published studies specifically on the effectiveness of efforts to increase awareness and knowledge of the interaction between TB and diabetes were identified. The guideline group's experts stressed that this recommendation should be an integral part of recommendations for training and capacity building on care of both conditions.

B.2. Ensure TB infection control in health-care settings where diabetes is managed

In diabetes clinics, where the risk of TB is higher than in the general population, the risk of transmitting TB is increased, and the consequence of transmission is more severe for a person with diabetes. Measures to reduce TB transmission have been identified in WHO's International Guidelines for TB infection Control, and include administrative and environmental control measures, which are aimed at generally reducing exposure to *Mycobacterium tuberculosis* for health-care workers and patients (*38*).

Administrative measures include early recognition, diagnosis and treatment of TB, particularly pulmonary TB, and separation of people with suspected pulmonary TB from others until a diagnosis is confirmed or excluded. Environmental protection should include maximizing natural ventilation with large, opened windows and doors, opening sky-lights for cross-ventilation and re-designing waiting rooms to be in the open air where possible (*39*). Mechanical ventilation systems should be considered where affordable, and, if used, regularly maintained.

Recommendation 9
Each health-care facility, including diabetes clinics, should have an infection control plan (including a plan for TB infection control), which includes administrative and environmental control measures to reduce transmission of TB within this setting. These measures should adhere to WHO's International Guidelines for TB infection Control.

Remark: The evidence for existing guidelines on TB infection control was not reviewed as part of the systematic review for this document. However, this recommendation is fully in line with existing guidelines on TB infection control (*38*).

B.3. Ensure high-quality treatment and management of TB in people with diabetes

Diabetes appears to impact negatively on the time to conversion of sputum culture, and is associated with an increased risk of death and increased risk of TB recurrence, although not recurrence caused by drug-resistant strains (*3*). The reasons for these adverse outcomes are not clear but may be associated with poor control of diabetes affecting TB treatment outcomes and drug–drug interactions.

Given the apparent increased vulnerability among people with diabetes, it is essential that all standard aspects of TB treatment and case management are optimized for this group. This includes correctly prescribed treatment regimens, optimal patient support and supervision, and clinical monitoring as per national guidelines and international standards. It also includes standard diagnosis, treatment and management of multidrug-resistant TB.

Currently, there is insufficient evidence to support changing the recommended standard TB treatment regimens or making specific recommendations for clinical case management of TB in people with diabetes. It is common clinical practice in some settings to extend the duration of TB treatment in people with diabetes. However, there are no published trials on the effectiveness of extending the duration of treatment.

Further research needs to be conducted to better understand drug–drug interactions and determine if any changes to drug choice and/or dosage are required.

There is not enough evidence to support any policy recommendation to give isoniazid preventive therapy, or any other preventive therapy, to diabetes patients with latent TB infection in order to prevent progression to active disease.

Recommendation 10
Treatment and case management of TB in people with diabetes should be provided in accordance with existing TB treatment guidelines and international standards. The same TB treatment regimen should be prescribed to people with diabetes as for people without diabetes.

Summary of assessment of graded evidence from the systematic reviews

Overall quality of evidence	Low
Balance of potential benefits and harms	Benefit
Disagreement among the panel	None
Acceptability	High
Feasibility	High
Resource implications	Moderate
Strength of recommendation	STRONG

Remark: There is evidence of low quality for a higher risk of delayed bacteriological conversion, and there is evidence of low to moderate quality for a higher risk of death and relapse among people with diabetes who are treated for TB, compared with TB patients without diabetes. This suggests that it is particularly important to ensure high-quality TB treatment according to existing standards in this group of patients. An extended period of TB treatment for people with diabetes has been suggested and is a recommended consideration in some settings (40). However, there are no published trials on the efficacy of extending the duration of TB treatment or other changes to the standard TB treatment regimens for people with diabetes. Therefore, the evidence on special TB treatment regimens for people with diabetes is low. There is evidence of low quality of no association between diabetes and drug-resistant TB. The guideline group's experts therefore agreed that there is no evidence to support special TB treatment regimens for people with diabetes. Patients should be treated according to existing guidelines on TB treatment until better evidence becomes available (23, 41).

C. Detect and manage diabetes in patients with Tuberculosis

C.1. Screen TB patients for diabetes

As discussed in section A.3. above, screening for diabetes among TB patients should be feasible in all countries where basic equipment and knowledge on diabetes is available in primary health-care settings. However, the best approach for screening, including timing and screening method used, has yet to be established. Further research should provide a clearer picture of the optimal method and timing of screening for diabetes in TB centres.

As an infectious disease, TB may temporarily elevate blood glucose levels and result in false-positive diagnoses of diabetes if investigations are performed too early. However, delayed screening may be a missed opportunity for early initiation of diabetes treatment and health education during the intensive phase of TB treatment, which potentially would have positive effects on both the management of diabetes and the results of TB treatment. Furthermore, hyperglycaemia, even if temporary, may be a risk factor for poor TB treatment outcomes. Testing at the time of diagnosis, in the TB diagnostic facility, may be advisable also for practical reasons. Many TB control programmes provide decentralized treatment to peripheral facilities where laboratory investigations are difficult to perform. Screening for diabetes is therefore recommended at the start of TB treatment, in the TB diagnostic centre, and to confirm the diabetes diagnosis as part of the clinical follow up of elevated blood glucose.

Operational and other research should be carried out to determine the best methods for diagnosing diabetes in TB patients, focusing on adults stratified by type of disease (smear-positive pulmonary TB, smear-negative pulmonary TB and extrapulmonary TB) and the most feasible and appropriate ways of screening.

Recommendation 11
TB patients should be screened for diabetes at the start of TB treatment, where resources for diagnosis are available. Type of screening and diagnostic tests should be adapted to the context of local health systems and the availability of resources, while awaiting additional evidence on the best screening and diagnostic approach.

Overall quality of evidence	Low
Balance of potential benefits and harms	Benefit
Disagreement among the panel	None
Acceptability	High
Feasibility	Dependent on setting
Resource implications	Low
Strength of recommendation	STRONG

Remark: The direct evidence for diabetes screening among people with TB is of low quality. Few published studies are available on the feasibility and additional yield of routine screening for diabetes among people with TB. There are no published studies on the impact of increased screening for diabetes among people with TB on morbidity or mortality from the disease. However, there is evidence of moderate quality that diabetes is associated with TB and that its prevalence among people with TB is two to three times higher than in the general population. Where diagnosis and treatment of diabetes is available and accessible, screening among TB patients should be considered as part of the basic clinical package. Existing guidelines for screening and diagnosis should be followed (*42*). Specific screening and diagnostic algorithms for diabetes among people with TB should be evaluated through research studies. Resource implications from a general health service perspective are judged to be low, since the number of TB patients to be screened is relatively small in most settings.

C.2. Ensure high-quality management of diabetes among TB patients

Care of diabetes is underdeveloped in many low-income and middle-income countries. Strengthening such services may be a necessary component of collaborative activities. Potentially, optimized care of diabetes among people with TB could be an entry point for improved care of the disease in the general health system. Although there are no published trials assessing if improved glucose control reduces the risk of adverse TB treatment outcomes, the existing evidence indirectly suggests that optimized management of diabetes in TB patients, including early diagnosis, optimized treatment and health education, and clinical and therapeutic monitoring, would improve TB treatment outcomes and reduce the risk of recurrent TB. Optimized diabetes management may also improve outcomes of other coinfections in diabetes, accounting for as much as 24% of deaths in African patients (*43*).

Further research needs to be conducted to better understand drug–drug interactions and determine if any changes to drug choice and/or dosage are required.

Recommendation 12
Management of diabetes in TB patients should be provided in line with existing guidelines.

Remark: The evidence for existing guidelines on management of diabetes was not reviewed as part of the systematic review for this document. However, this recommendation is in line with existing guidelines on management of the disease, including special considerations for people with worsened glucose control as an effect of an ongoing infection (*44–46*).

4. Indicators for evaluating collaborative activities

Monitoring a set of key process and outcome indicators would enable countries, organizations and institutions to work towards common goals, and help to accelerate country-level implementation of collaborative activities. The proposed indicators listed below may be monitored at clinic, district, province and/or national levels. The choice among these indicators, and possible additional indicators, depends on the local scope of collaborative TB and diabetes activities.

Careful monitoring of these indicators would also be the basis for operational research on the feasibility, effectiveness and cost-effectiveness of different models of collaboration. Such operational research, which should ideally also include qualitative research methods, will be a crucial complement to clinical studies when addressing the research questions listed in Annex II.

Proposed indicators
1. Joint TB and diabetes plan in place (Y/N)
2. Number and proportion of people with diagnosed diabetes that have been screened for chronic cough.
3. Number and proportion of people with diagnosed diabetes that have been tested for TB (radiography, sputum smear microscopy, culture, etc).
4. Prevalence of TB among people with diabetes.
5. Number and proportion of people with TB that have been screened for diabetes.
6. Prevalence of diabetes among people with TB.
7. TB treatment outcomes among people with diabetes.

5. Implementing collaborative activities and evaluating their impact

The first set of recommendations in this framework concerns mechanisms for collaboration, and suggests how stakeholders should work together to ensure optimal coordination and local adaptation, and how to monitor progress using the indicators suggested in section 4 (see sections 3A and 4). The recommendation to set up joint coordination involves identification of barriers and facilitating factors for implementation as well as local adaptation of the recommendations contained in sections 3B and 3C, which should translate into specific national guidance within plans for diabetes and TB care and prevention respectively.

The framework will be disseminated through WHO regional and country offices to Ministries of Health and relevant public health programmes, as well as national and international partners involved in prevention and care of both diseases. The Union, the International Diabetes Federation and other technical agencies working in partnership with WHO will disseminate the framework through their respective networks.

Regular and joint evaluation of the guideline's quality, usefulness and impact will be done by WHO, the Union, the International Diabetes Federation and other partners.

Annex I. Members of the Guideline Group

Expert	Professional affiliation	Area of expertise
Professor Mauricio Barreto	Instituto de Saude Coletiva, Universidade Federal da Bahia, Bahia, Brazil	DM and TB research and epidemiology
Dr Meghan A Baker	Department of Epidemiology, Harvard School of Public Health, Boston, MA, US	TB and DM researcher, performed the systematic review
Dr Nils Billo	International Union against Tuberculosis and Lung Disease, Paris, France	TB and public health expert
Dr Richard Brostrom	US Centers for Disease Control and Prevention, Regional Field Medical Officer, US Pacific Region, Hawaii State TB Controller	US CDC representative. TB and DM clinician and epidemiologist. Developer of Pacific TB and Diabetes Guidelines.
Professor Ib Christian Bygbjerg	Department of International Health, Immunology and Microbiology, University of Copenhagen, Denmark	Global Health expert; TB and DM research; TB clinical practice
Dr Martin Castellanos	Centro Nacional de Vigilancia Epidemiológica y Control de Enfermedades, Mexico City, Mexico	TB programme planner and implementer, Mexico. TB research
Dr Saidi Egwaga	National Tuberculosis and Leprosy Programme, Dar-es-Salaam, United Republic of Tanzania	TB programme planner and implementer, United Republic of Tanzania. TB research
Professor Susan Fisher-Hoch	School of Public Health, University of Texas Health Science Center, Houston, USA	TB research in Africa and Asia. DM in disadvantaged populations and associations between DM & TB.
Professor Anthony D. Harries	International Union against Tuberculosis and Lung Disease, Paris, France [2] London School of Hygiene and Tropical Medicine, Keppel Street, London, UK	TB, HIV, and DM research and clinical practice
Dr Christie Y Jeon	Center for Infectious Disease Epidemiologic Research, Mailman School of Public Health, Columbia University, New York, NY, U.S.	TB and DM research, performed the systematic review

Dr Knut Lönnroth	Stop-TB Department, World Health Organization, Geneva, Switzerland	TB epidemiology; research on TB risk factors and co-morbidities; health systems research
Professor Megan B. Murray	Department of Epidemiology, Harvard School of Public Health, Boston, MA, US Division of Global Health Equity, Brigham & Women's Hospital, Boston, MA, US	TB and DM research and epidemiology, performed the systematic review
Dr Toru Mori	Research Institute of Tuberculosis, Kiyose, Tokyo, Japan	TB research and epidemiology; TB programme planner and implementer, Japan
Dr Salah-Eddine Ottmani	Stop-TB Department, World Health Organization, Geneva, Switzerland	TB epidemiology; research on TB risk factors and co-morbidities
Dr Kaushik Ramaiya	Shree Hindu Mandal Hospital, Dar Es Salaam, United Republic of Tanzania; Department of Medicine, Muhimbili University of Health and Allied Sciences, Dar Es Salaam, United Republic of Tanzania	TB and DM research and clinical practice, Hon General Secretary of Association of Private Health Facilities in Tanzania. Hon General Secretary, Tanzania Diabetes Association
Dr Gojka Roglic	Department of Chronic Diseases and Health Promotion, World Health Organization, Geneva, Switzerland	DM research and epidemiology
Professor Nigel Unwin	Faculty of Medical Sciences, Cave Hill Campus, University of the West Indies	DM and TB research and epidemiology
Dr Vijay Viswanathan	M.V.Hospital for Diabetes and Research Centre, Royapuram, Chennai, India	TB and DM research and epidemiology
Dr David Whiting	International Diabetes Federation, Brussels, Belgium	DM epidemiology and research, representative of International Diabetes Federation
Dr Lixia Wang	National Center for TB Control and Prevention, China Centers for Disease Control, Beijing, China	TB programme planner and implementer, China
Dr Wenhua Zhao	National Center for Chronic Disease control and Prevention China Centers for Disease Control, Beijing, China	NCD programme planner and implementer, China

Annex II. Summary grading of the evidence[1]

No. of Studies	Design	Quality assessment					Summary of findings			Importance
		Limitations	Inconsistency	Indirectness	Imprecision	Other considerations	Effect	Absolute	Quality	
Is diabetes associated with TB infection? (see support material 1 at http://www.who.int/tb/publications/2011/en/index.html)										
4	Cross-sectional studies	Serious limitations	Consistent no association	Serious	Serious	None	1.01 (0.78, 1.31)	N/A	Low	Moderately important
Is diabetes associated with active TB disease? (see support material 1 at http://www.who.int/tb/publications/2011/en/index.html)										
4	Cohort studies	Some limitations	Consistent positive associations, with large heterogeneity	Serious	Moderately serious	None	2.52 (1.53, 4.03)	N/A	Moderate	Important
10	Case-control studies	Some limitations	Mostly positive associations, with large heterogeneity	Moderately serious	Moderately serious	None	2.20 (1.78, 2.73)	N/A	Low-Moderate	
Is diabetes associated with positive sputum culture at 2-3 months? (see support material 2 at http://www.who.int/tb/publications/2011/en/index.html)										
8	Observational studies	Some limitations	Mostly positive associations, with large heterogeneity	Moderately serious	Serious	None	RR range 0.79 to 3.25	N/A	Low	Moderately important
Is diabetes associated with favourable treatment outcome? (see support material 2 at http://www.who.int/tb/publications/2011/en/index.html)										
13	Observational studies	Serious limitations	Mostly null findings with large heterogeneity	Serious	Not Serious	None	0.95 (0.91, 0.98)	N/A	Very Low	Important

[1] Support material on the web (http://www.who.int/tb/publications/2011/en/index.html) include detailed summary tables of all reviewed studies and indicate for each question the annex in which the details of the studies are included.

colspan="8"	**Is diabetes associated with death during treatment period?** (see support material 2 at http://www.who.int/tb/publications/2011/en/index.html)
23	Observational studies with no adjustment for confounders	Serious limitations	Mostly positive associations, with large heterogeneity	Serious	Moderately serious	None	1.85 (1.50, 2.28)	N/A	Low	Important
4	Observational studies with adjustment for confounders	Some limitations	Consistent positive associations	Serious	Serious	None	4.95 (2.69, 9.10)	N/A	Moderate	
colspan="8"	**Is diabetes associated with relapse?** (see support material 2 at http://www.who.int/tb/publications/2011/en/index.html)
4	Observational studies	Some limitations	Consistent positive associations	Moderately serious	Serious	None	3.98 (2.11, 7.50)	N/A	Moderate	Important
colspan="8"	**Is diabetes associated with drug-resistance?** (see support material 2 at http://www.who.int/tb/publications/2011/en/index.html)
3	Observational studies on primary DR TB (any DR TB)	Some limitations	Consistent no association	Serious	Serious	None	1.01 (0.63, 1.63)	N/A	Low	Important
2	Observational studies on acquired DR TB	Some limitations	Consistent no association	Serious	Serious	None	0.86 (0.39, 1.88)	N/A	Low	
4	Observational studies on any DR TB without distinction of primary or acquired	Serious Limitations	Consistent no association	Serious	Serious	None	1.02 (0.70, 1.49)	N/A	Very Low	
2	Observational studies on primary MDR TB	Some limitations	Consistent positive association	Serious	Serious	None	2.91 (1.26, 6.72)	N/A	Low	
1	Observational studies on acquired MDR TB	Some limitations	No association	Serious	Serious	Small power	0.8 (0.2, 4.2)	N/A	Low	
9	Observational studies on MDR TB without distinction of primary or acquired	Serious Limitations	Inconsistent	Moderately serious	Moderately serious	None	1.86 (1.39, 2.50)	N/A	Very Low	
1	Observational studies on XDR TB	Some limitations	No association	Serious	Serious	Small power	2.1 (0.64, 6.9)	N/A	Low	

Does screening for DM among TB lead to more TB case detection? (see support material 3 at http://www.who.int/tb/publications/2011/en/index.html)								
10	Observational studies on screening for prevalent TB in DM	Serious limitations	Large heterogeneity, but consistently greater TB prevalence than in comparison	Moderately serious	Serious	Some studies lack control group	TB prevalence in DM higher than in comparison, where available	N/A	Very Low	Important
2	Observational studies on screening for incident TB in DM	Serious limitations	Large heterogeneity, but consistently greater TB incidence than in comparison	Serious	Serious	Some studies lack control group	TB incidence in DM higher than in comparison, where available	N/A	Very Low	
5	Observational studies on screening for prevalent TB infection in DM	Serious limitations	Some heterogeneity, but mostly similar TB infection prevalence as in comparison	Serious	Serious	Some studies lack control group	TB infection prevalence in DM similar to comparison population, where available	N/A	Very Low	Moderately important
Does screening for DM among TB patients lead to more DM detection? (see support material 3 at http://www.who.int/tb/publications/2011/en/index.html)								
7	Observational studies on screening for DM after TB Tx initiation	Serious limitations	Some heterogeneity, but generally greater DM prevalence than in comparison	Moderately serious	Serious	Some studies lack control group	DM prevalence in TB higher than in comparison, where available	N/A	Low	Important
11	Observational studies on screening for DM before TB Tx initiation, or timing unclear	Serious limitations	Large heterogeneity, but generally greater DM prevalence than in comparison	Moderately serious	Serious	Some studies lack control group	DM prevalence in TB higher than in comparison, where available	N/A	Very Low	
Does hyperglycaemia initially found in TB patients resolve with TB treatment? (see support material 3 at http://www.who.int/tb/publications/2011/en/index.html)								
4	Observational studies on screening with multiple follow-up	Serious limitations	Consistent	Serious	Serious	No control groups	Prevalence of hyperglycaemia decreases with TB treatment	N/A	Low	Important

2	Observational studies	Serious limitations	Consistent		Studies lacked crucial details on study design and findings	Both report reduced TB incidence	N/A	Very Low	Moderately important

Is chemoprophylaxis intervention in DM effective in preventing TB? (see support material 3 at http://www.who.int/tb/publications/2011/en/index.html)

Does screening for TB among DM lead to prevention of TB morbidity and mortality than not screening?

no study

Does screening for DM among TB lead to prevention of DM morbidity and mortality than not screening?

no study

DM = diabetes mellitus; TB = tuberculosis; Tx = treatment

Annex III. Key research questions for improving the prevention, management and care of diabetes and tuberculosis *(31)*

Key research questions	Priority	Study design and methodology
Screening for Disease: • Screening patients with DM for active TB • Screening patients with TB for DM	High	Prospective observational cohort studies of DM patients routinely attending diabetic clinics and screened for TB, and TB patients starting anti-TB treatment and screened for diabetes
TB treatment outcomes in patients with DM, including a more detailed assessment of death during anti-TB treatment	High	Prospective observational cohort studies using standardized TB regimens and standardized treatment outcomes and focusing on defined primary outcomes Prospective observational cohort studies determining when death occurs in relation to start of TB treatment, the etiology and whether case fatality is reduced by better DM control
Implementing and evaluating the "DOTS" model for standardized case management of DM	High	Operational research including quarterly cohort reporting of new cases, treatment outcomes of cumulative cases including frequency of co-morbidities such as TB, and survival analysis
Development and evaluation of a point of care glycated haemoglobin test (HbA1c)	High	Developmental work to develop a dipstick for measuring HbA1c for use in rural areas, which then needs to be tested for efficacy and feasibility in the field
Rates of hospitalization and additional medical costs associated with diagnosis and management of dual disease	Medium	Cross-sectional studies
Use of the community to improve management and care of patients with DM and TB	Medium	Operational research
Household contact tracing of adult patients with smear-positive pulmonary TB	Medium	Prospective observational studies to determine the yield of screening household contacts for TB infection, active TB, HIV and DM, and to assess whether DM influences the establishment of TB infection
Radiographic findings in DM patients with TB	Medium	Systematic review of the literature and prospective cross-sectional studies if further evidence is required to determine the common radiographic patterns
Modelling the effect of the DM epidemic on the TB epidemic	Medium	Mathematical modelling studies
TB preventive therapy in patients with DM	Low	Randomized controlled trial assessing efficacy and safety of isoniazid preventive therapy in reducing risk of active TB in patients with DM

DM = diabetes mellitus; HIV = human immunodeficiency virus; TB = tuberculosis

References

1. Lönnroth K et al. Tuberculosis control and elimination 2010–50: cure, care, and social development. *Lancet*, 2010, 375:1814–1829.

2. Jeon CY, Murray MB. Diabetes mellitus increases the risk of active tuberculosis: a systematic review of 13 observational studies. *PLoS Medicine*, 2008, 5:e152.

3. Baker MA et al. Systematic review: the impact of diabetes on tuberculosis treatment outcomes BMC Medicine accepted 2011, 9: 81.

4. Goldhaber-Fiebert JD et al. Diabetes mellitus and tuberculosis in countries with high tuberculosis burdens: individual risks and social determinants. *International Journal of Epidemiology*, 2011, 40:417–428.

5. Dye C et al. Nutrition, Diabetes and Tuberculosis in the Epidemiological Transition. *PLoS ONE*, 2011, 6(6):e21161 (doi:10.1371/journal.pone.0021161).

6. Shaw J, Sicree R, Zimmet P. Global estimates of the prevalence of diabetes for 2010 and 2030. *Diabetes Research and Clinical Practice*, 2010, 87:4–14.

7. Roglic G, Unwin N. Mortality attributable to diabetes: estimates for the year 2010. *Diabetes Research and Clinical Practice*, 2010, 87:15–19.

8. Wild S et al. Global prevalence of diabetes: estimates for the year 2000 and projections for 2030. *Diabetes Care*, 2004, 27:1047–1053.

9. Whiting D, Unwin N, Roglic G. Diabetes: equity and social determinants. In: Blas E, Sivasankara Kurup A, eds. *Priority public health conditions: from learning to action on social determinants of health.* Geneva, World Health Organization, 2010 (pp77-94).

10. Blas E, Sivasankara Kurup A, eds. *Priority public health conditions: from learning to action on social determinants of health.* Geneva, World Health Organization, 2010.

11. Restrepo BI. Convergence of the tuberculosis and diabetes epidemics: renewal of old acquaintances. *Clinical Infectious Diseases*, 2007, 45:436–438.

12. Dooley KE, Chaisson RE. Tuberculosis and diabetes mellitus: convergence of two epidemics. *Lancet Infectious Diseases*, 2009; 9:737–746.

13. Brock I et al. Latent tuberculosis in HIV positive, diagnosed by the *M. tuberculosis* specific interferon-gamma test. *Respiratory Research*, 2006, 7:56.

14. Chan-Yeung M et al. Prevalence and determinants of positive tuberculin reactions of residents in old age homes in Hong Kong. *International Journal of Tuberculosis and Lung Disease*, 2006, 10:892–898.

15. Stevenson CR et al. Diabetes and the risk of tuberculosis: a neglected threat to public health? *Chronic Illness*, 2007, 3:228–245.

16. Stevenson CR et al. Diabetes and tuberculosis: the impact of the diabetes epidemic on tuberculosis incidence. *BMC Public Health*, 2007, 7:234.

17. Fisher-Hoch SP et al. Type 2 diabetes and multidrug-resistant tuberculosis. *Scandinavian Journal of Infectious Diseases*, 2008, 40:888–893.

18. Nijland HM et al. Exposure to rifampicin is strongly reduced in patients with tuberculosis and type 2 diabetes. *Clinical Infectious Diseases*, 2006, 43:848–854.

19. *Global tuberculosis control: WHO report 2010*. Geneva, World Health Organization, 2010 (WHO/HTM/TB/2010.7).

20. Storla DG, Yimer S, Bjune GA. A systematic review of delay in the diagnosis and treatment of tuberculosis. *BMC Public Health*, 2008, 8:15.

21. Lonnroth K et al. Drivers of tuberculosis epidemics: the role of risk factors and social determinants. *Social Science & Medicine*, 2009, 68:2240–2246.

22. Raviglione MC, Uplekar M. WHO's new Stop TB Strategy. *Lancet*, 2006, 367: 952–955.

23. Hopewell PC et al. International Standards for Tuberculosis Care. *Lancet Infectious Diseases*, 2006, 6:710–725.

24. *Preventing chronic diseases: a vital investment*. Geneva, World Health Organization, 2005.

25. *A WHO/The Union monograph on TB and tobacco control*. Geneva, World Health Organization, 2008 (WHO/TB/2007.390).

26. *Scoping meeting for the development of guidelines on nutritional/food support to prevent TB and improve health status among TB patients*. Geneva, World Health Organization, 2009.

27. Lönnroth K et al. Alcohol use as a risk factor for tuberculosis – a systematic review. *BMC Public Health*, 2008, 8:289.

28. *Policy guidelines for collaborative TB and HIV services for injecting and other drug users: an integrated approach.* Geneva, World Health Organization, 2008 (WHO/HTM/TB/2008.404).

29. *Handbook for guideline development.* Geneva, World Health Organization, 2010.

30. Ottmani SE et al. Consultation meeting on tuberculosis and diabetes mellitus: meeting summary and recommendations. *International Journal of Tuberculosis and Lung Disease*, 2010, 14:1513–1517.

31. Harries AD et al. Defining the research agenda to reduce the joint burden of disease from Diabetes mellitus and Tuberculosis. *Tropical Medicine & International Health*, 2010,15:659–663.

32. Feigenbaum K, Longstaff L. Management of the metabolic syndrome in patients with human immunodeficiency virus. *The Diabetes Educator*, 2010, 36(3):457–464.

33. Jeon CY et al. Bi-directional screening for tuberculosis and diabetes: a systematic review. *Tropical Medicine & International Health*, 2010, 15:1300–1314.

34. *Use of glycated haemoglobin (HbA1c) in the diagnosis of diabetes mellitus..* Geneva, World Health Organization, 2011 (WHO/NMH/CHP/CPM/11.1).

35. Harries AD, Billo N, Kapur A. Links between diabetes mellitus and tuberculosis: should we integrate screening and care? *Transactions of the Royal Society of Tropical Medicine and Hygiene*, 2009, 103:1–2.

36. Harries AD et al. Adapting the DOTS framework for tuberculosis control to the management of non-communicable diseases in sub-Saharan Africa. *PLoS Medicine*, 2008, 5:e124.

37. *Implementing the WHO Stop TB Strategy.* Geneva, World Health Organization, 2010 (WHO/HTM/TB/2008.401).

38. *WHO policy on TB infection control in health-care facilities, congregate settings and households.* Geneva, World Health Organization, 2009 (WHO/HTM/TB/2009.419).

39. Escombe AR et al. Natural ventilation for the prevention of airborne contagion. *PLoS Medicine*, 2007, 4:e68.

40. *Draft Interim U.S. Associated Pacific Islands (USAPI) Standards for the management of tuberculosis and diabetes*. Agana, Guam, Pacific Island Tuberculosis Controllers Association, 2011 (available at: http://www.nationaltbcenter.edu/abouttb/TB_DM_USAPI_Standards_document_12_01_2010.pdf).

41. *Treatment of tuberculosis: guidelines*, 4th ed. Geneva, World Health Organization, 2010 (WHO/HTM/TB/2009.420).

42. *Definition and diagnosis of diabetes mellitus and intermediate hyperglycaemia: report of a WHO/IDF consultation*. Geneva, World Health Organization, 2006.

43. McLarty DG, Kinabo L, Swai AB. Diabetes in tropical Africa: a prospective study, 1981-7. II. Course and prognosis. *BMJ*, 1990, 300:1107–1110.

44. National Collaborating Centre for Chronic Conditions. *Type 2 diabetes: national clinical guideline for management in primary and secondary care* [update]. London, Royal College of Physicians, 2008.

45. *Global guideline for type 2 diabetes*. Brussels, International Diabetes Federation, 2005.

46. *Type 1 diabetes: diagnosis and management of type 1 diabetes in children, young people and adults*. London: National Institute for Clinical Excellence, 2004 (available at: www.nice.org.uk/CG015NICEguideline).